T0197445

The Magical Stickers

Darlene Louf

AuthorHouse™
1663 Liberty Drive
Bloomington, IN 47403
www.authorhouse.com
Phone: 833-262-8899

Because of the dynamic nature of the Internet, any web addresses or links contained in this book may have changed
since publication and may no longer be valid. The views expressed in this work are solely those of the author and do not
necessarily reflect the views of the publisher, and the publisher hereby disclaims any responsibility for them.

Any people depicted in stock imagery provided by Getty Images are models,
and such images are being used for illustrative purposes only.
Certain stock imagery © Getty Images.

This book is printed on acid-free paper.

ISBN: 978-1-5462-0438-1 (sc)
ISBN: 978-1-5462-0439-8 (e)

Library of Congress Control Number: 2017912637

Print information available on the last page.

Published by AuthorHouse 09/20/2022

authorHOUSE®

This story based on real life events was written to help families explain the diagnosis of cancer to their children or grandchildren. I am hoping that this book will make things easier for children to understand and cope with a diagnosis of cancer in the family.

The Magical Stickers is dedicated to: my grandson Kyle Wilson and my children Angie Saulnier and Jeremiah Louf.

Thank you for all your love and support.

The Magical Stickers book is in memory of all who have lost their battles to cancer.

At four and a half years old Kyle is very energetic and loved to spend time with his Grammy. You could find him with her up to three times a week. To Kyle this was the best part of his week. He loved trips to the park and shopping trips. If they went to the dollar store Grammy would always give him a dollar to buy anything he wanted. On days when the weather was bad they would stay at Grammy's and watch TV. It was usually Sesame Street; Kyle's favorite Character was Elmo. No matter what they were doing they always loved spending time together.

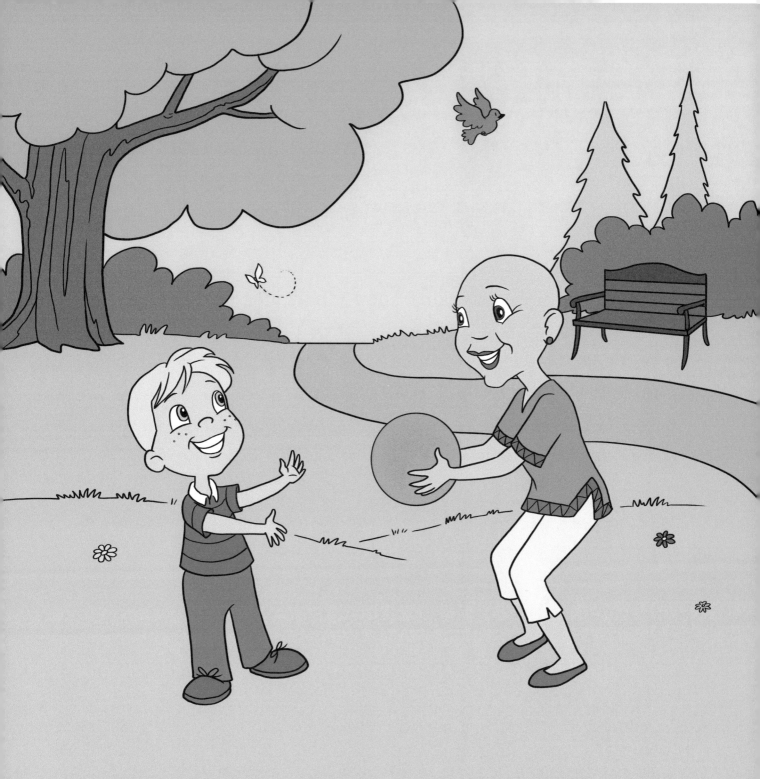

Suddenly Grammy couldn't see Kyle as often and he was upset. She became sick and was in a lot of pain. She thought she had a bad cold, so she went to see her doctor. After describing how she felt; the doctor put Kyle's Grammy in the hospital to run some tests. He was hoping the test would allow them to see why she didn't feel good. Grammy told the doctor that she had a really bad stomach ache. But she didn't know why she had it. And it lasted a long time. The doctor put her in the hospital for five very long days.

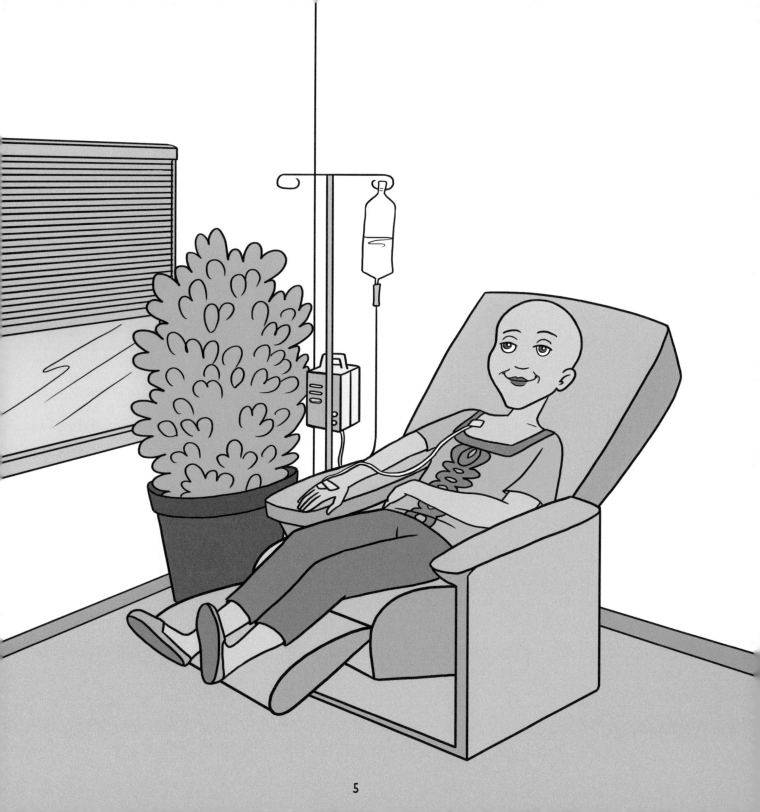

After many tests the doctor told Grammy that she had breast cancer and a blood clot in her kidney. That was why Kyle couldn't see her as often. It was making him really sad.

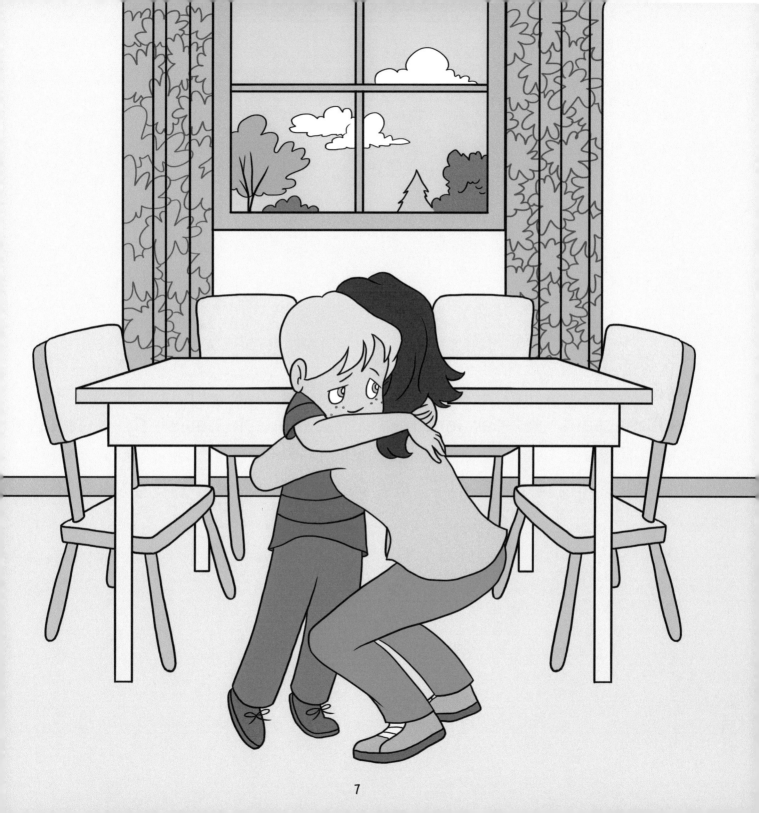

Kyle's Mommy explained to him that Grammy was very sick. She showed him a TV show called Arthur where one of the characters had cancer. The show made it easier for Kyle to understand what was going on with Grammy. It also helped him understand why he didn't see Grammy as much as he used to.

When Grammy was feeling better the doctor let her go home. She had to start taking a special cancer medicine called Chemotherapy. It is a very strong medicine that would help Grammy get better. The doctor put a special device in her called a port-a-cath.

This special device was placed under the skin on the left side of Grammy's chest. It was used to give Grammy her special medicine. The doctor told Grammy it was the safest and easiest way to get her medicine.

Grammy's long road to fighting cancer began. She explained to Kyle that that the medicine would help her, but she may loose her hair. Grammy did loose all her hair. She needed to wear wigs and scarves when she went out. But it was hard to wear them because her medicine made her head and body sore. Most of the time she couldn't wear wigs or scarves because they hurt her head. This made her upset because she couldn't see Kyle as much as she wanted to. She was afraid that him seeing her without hair would be scary.

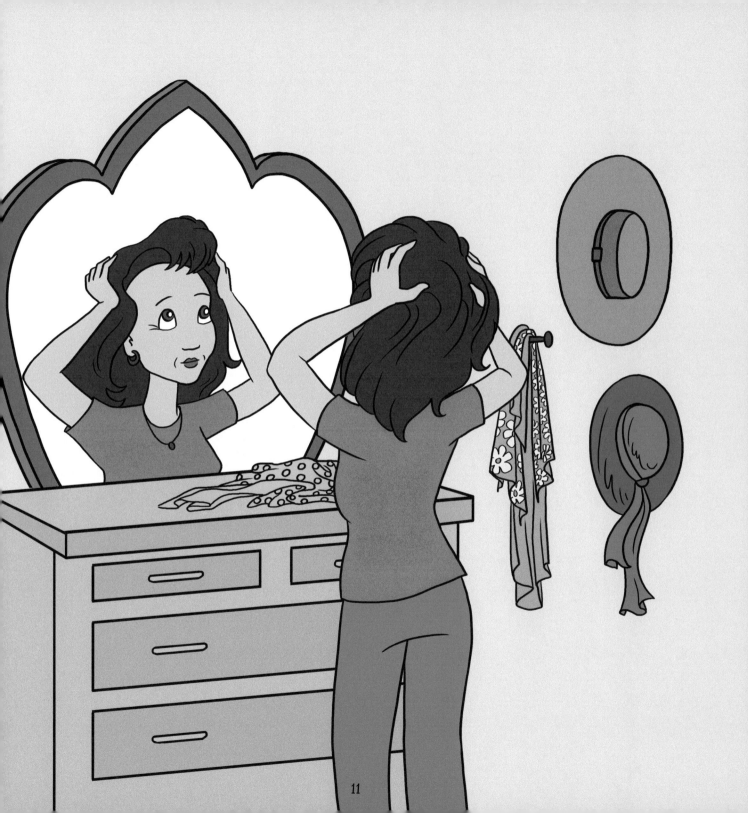

Then Grammy had an idea. She thought of a very special way to explain everything to Kyle. She wanted Kyle to be comfortable and not to be scared because she didn't have any hair. That way she could start spending time with him again. Grammy knew Kyle loved doing crafts and stickers. Grammy went to Kyle's favorite store and bought 500 stickers. There were so many stickers! Some had smiley faces and even some of Kyle's favorite Sesame Street Characters.

One day Kyle came home from school and grammy was sitting at the kitchen table. He was happy to see her that a hug smile came across his face. He gave her a great big hug! Suddenly he backed up looking very confused. For the first time since grammy got sick he saw her wearing a pretty scarf on her head, but there was no hair. Kyle was very surprised.

Grammy said, "Kyle, you know grammy has been sick for a while with cancer? Well because of the special medicine they are giving me I am losing my hair. That's why I am wearing this pretty scarf".

He turned his head and looked at his mommy and then back to his grammy. Grammy said "Kyle are you ok"? Kyle smiled and said, "yes grammy i am ok"! Grammy said, "I need your help". Kyle quickly responded "what can I do grammy"? Grammy explained, "when I take off this scarf I won't have any hair and I don't want you to be scared". Grammy then removed the scarf. Kyle backed up and looked at grammy. But, "grammy I am a little scared" Kyle said softly. Grammy said, "it's of Kyle, would you like to touch it"? Kyle looked at his mommy and she nodded and said, it's ok Kyle. Kyle then looked at his grammy again and reached over and touched her head.

He made a funny face and said

"YUCK! It feels like daddy's face when he does not shave!" Everyone laughed a lot. Grammy showed Kyle the stickers she bought him.

She then said, "Grammy needs your help. If you take these stickers and put them all over my head my hair will grow back. Would you be a special part of my recovery?" A huge smile grew on Kyle's face and with joy in his voice he replied "Yes Grammy I would!"

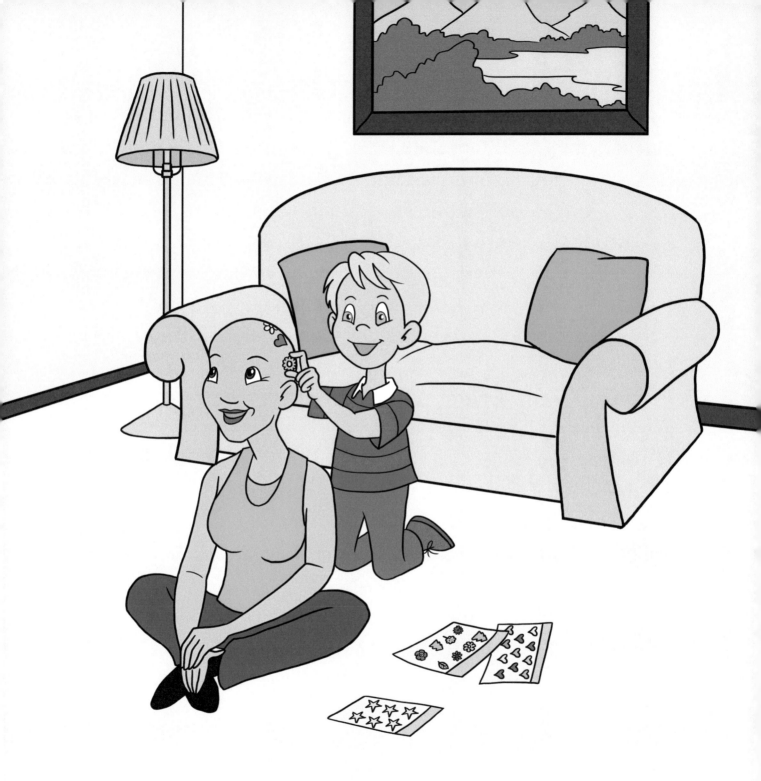

Kyle sat Grammy on the floor and he began putting the stickers all over her head. Together they laughed and just enjoyed each other's company. All of a sudden Kyle was no longer afraid of his Grammy's baldhead. He put all 500 stickers on her head. He thought Grammy looked a little funny, but wanted her to get better. They both laughed and laughed. Grammy had 500 stickers on her head. When he finally finished Grammy said

   "Kyle the magic of your love is going to help my hair grow back"

He replied with "Grammy don't take them off until all your hair grows back."

"I will do my best Kyle, but they may fall off when I take a shower. But if they do I will put them back on for you! Ok?" Grammy answered.

Kyle happily responded "Ok Grammy! Do you want to play with my toys?"

Together they began to play. For the rest of the day Grammy left the stickers on her head. Kyle understood that that there are times that Grammy couldn't wear a wig or scarf because they hurt her head. He wasn't afraid anymore!

A few weeks later Grammy took Kyle for one of their special visits. She was wearing a wig and it was bothering her head. Grammy asked Kyle if she could take off the wig. Kyle looked at Grammy with love in his eyes and said

"It is ok Grammy go ahead."

She thanked him as she took off her wig. She starting rubbing her head and explained to Kyle that it hurt where she was rubbing. Kyle looked at the spot she was pointing to and said "Silly Grammy your wig is too tight."

They both laughed and Kyle told her she didn't need to put her wig back on.

Then one day Grammy's hair began to grow back. It was very short, soft, and looked like a baby's head. Grammy was so excited! She went with Kyle's Mommy to pick him up at school and take him out for ice cream. That way they could share the good news with him. Kyle came home from school and got into Grammy's car. With excitement Grammy said "Kyle remember when you put all those stickers on my head?"

"Yes Grammy I do." Kyle responded

She then said, "Those stickers had magic and with your special love something wonderful happened. Remember how I told you that if you put them all over my head my hair would grow back? And that you would play a big part in my recovery?"

Kyle answered "Yes Grammy I do!"

"Ok Kyle on the count of three I'm going to take my wig off" Grammy Explained

"1"

"2"

"3"

Grammy took her wig off and Kyle jumped out of his seat with such joy. He kept shouting

"Oh my goodness Oh my goodness. Grammy your hair is growing back!" he said it with such joy and excitement.

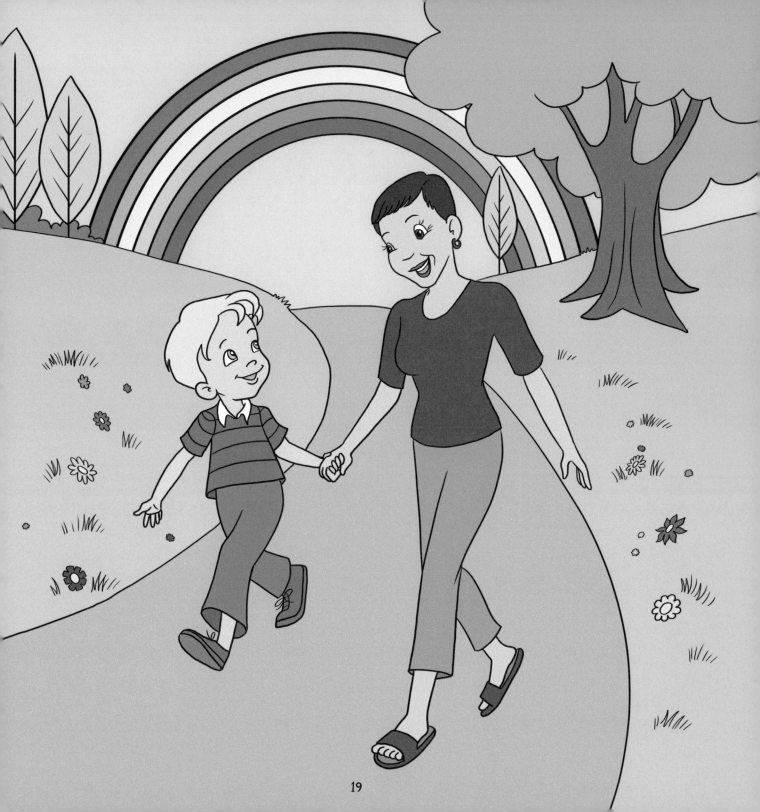

Grammy and his Mommy both began to cry tears of joy. Kyle then jumped to the front seat of the car and gave his Grammy the biggest hug he could. As Grammy hugged him back she said "This all happened because of the magic stickers and all the love you gave to Grammy.

Kyle and his Grammy knew from that day forward everything was going to be ok!

Printed in the United States
by Baker & Taylor Publisher Services